G000123193

NATURE'S PHARMACY

a guide to medicinal herbs

Deborah Fowler

Halzephron Herb Farm

First published in 2004 by Truran, Croft Prince, Mount Hawke, Truro,
Cornwall TR4 8EE
www.Truranbooks.co.uk
Truran is an imprint of Truran Books Ltd

Reprinted 2005

Cover image courtesy of Comstock from Cadmium Royalty Free

ISBN 1 85022 189 8

Printed and bound in Cornwall by R Booth Ld,
Antron Hill, Mabe, Penryn, Cornwall TR10 9HH

For Granny Ada, in loving memory

CONTENTS

INTRODUCTION

My Grandmother was a kleptomaniac. It did not matter whose garden we visited – friend or foe – the moment everyone's back was turned, out would come a rather elegant pair of nail scissors – a snip here, a snip there, and tiny cuttings would go into a paper bag she kept in her pocket as the repository for her booty. She was shameless. She took cuttings from Hampton Court, Blenheim Palace, Windsor Castle – even the illustrious Kew Gardens – and I was happy to play Oliver to her Artful Dodger.

My Granny's criminal activities are responsible for my own love of gardening, and it is from her that I first glimpsed the power of plant healing. As well as being asked to fetch rosemary for the leg of lamb she was cooking, likely as not, she would send me to find comfrey leaves over which she would pour boiling water to make a poultice for a bruise, or dandelion leaves to bind a wart. She had bottle upon bottle of tinctures – all gin based – which my father reckoned was just her way of providing the excuse for a tipple each evening! She had a medicine for every occasion, and from a child's perspective, it seemed to me then that she could cure anything. Perhaps she could.

When I started Halzephron Herb Farm and began developing my own range of herbal medicines I wished – and still do – that I had paid more attention to my Granny's recipes and knowledge.

From the mid 1900s, the increasing use of antibiotics – while very marvellous in their way – eclipsed all other forms of healing. My Grandmother's way of life seemed to have gone forever. From then until very recently, attitudes to illness appear to have developed along the lines that you wait until you are ill and then attempt to knock the illness on the head with a large dose of prescription drugs. Now, people are rediscovering alternative methods of healing, preventative medicine, aimed at arming the body to fight off infection and disease. Herbal medicines work WITH the body, not AGAINST it. Herbal remedies are nothing new – they have been with us for thousands of years. This book provides an opportunity to relearn what our forebears took for granted – LETTING NATURE HELP YOU TO HELP YOURSELF.

Deborah Fowler, Cornwall

HERBAL PREPARATIONS
how to use them

It would be irresponsible to begin this book without a word of warning. While I believe passionately in the value of medicinal herbs, it is important that their place is recognised alongside conventional medicine and, indeed, other alternative healing methods. Serious medical conditions should always be referred to your doctor and you should not suspend the taking of regular prescription medicines without first seeking medical advice. However, in today's hectic world, the poor beleaguered GP often cannot give enough attention to the common recurring ailments from which we all suffer, and which on the face of it – because they are not life threatening – can often be dismissed as trivial. For example – back pain, tinnitus, eczema, stress, the menopause, acne, insomnia – horrible for the sufferers, affecting every aspect of their lives, yet often either not taken seriously, or, in some cases, over medicated with drugs which create their own set of problems.

However, because I am stressing the use of medicinal herbs for non-chronic illness, please do not feel I am trying to trivialise their use. They have a very vital role to play in the most serious of illnesses, often working alongside traditional treatment. For example, take liver cancer – after a debilitating course of chemotherapy, milk thistle helps the liver to rejuvenate itself. There are herbs, such as garlic and hawthorn berry which help prevent heart disease, and herbs such as ginkgo leaf which is a sort of brain tonic, helping prevent strokes and thrombosis, while at the same time easing the suffering of chronic illnesses such as multiple sclerosis and dementia. The point I am trying to make, is that conventional medicine and herbal medicine can often be very compatible when used together, even for chronic illness.

It is equally important to stress that herbal medicine should not be seen simply as a substitute for the 'real thing'. In many instances, herbal medicine can be the better medicine to choose. In our increasingly nanny state, mercifully, we are still allowed to make decisions about our own bodies, and if you find a herbal medicine that particularly suits your needs then you are free to choose it, and use it.

Most of the herbs that I will be describing in this book can be bought in tablet form, over the counter. The alternative, of course, is that you grow the herbs yourself, and this can be very rewarding. The best herbs are organic herbs and this is something you can control if you do your own growing. Of course, some herbs are difficult to grow in this country, and some are impossible. However, many of the traditional remedies for healing are based on plants which have grown in our hedgerows for centuries, so many medicinal herbs are extremely easy to grow because they are indigenous to our countryside. If you are growing your own herbs for the purpose of healing, it is very important that you pick only the most perfect leaves/flowers/roots or berries. Always try to pick your herbs first thing in the morning and follow the seasons. Leaves are best picked in the spring when the sap has risen, roots and bark are best in the autumn when the goodness from the leaves has been passed into them, while clearly fruit should be picked as it comes to ripeness. The fresher and healthier the plant, the more good it will do you.

Preparations

If you are planning to prepare your own medications, this can be done from fresh or dried herbs and there are several methods for extracting the goodness. The main methods are either infusion or decoction – infusion in the case of soft plant parts – ie flowers and leaves, and decoction in the case of bark, seeds, and roots, from which the properties are more difficult to extract.

Infusion

Use 30g (1oz) of dried herbs or 75g (2½oz) of freshly chopped herbs to every 500ml (17½ fl oz) of water. Place the herbs in a teapot and pour over water which has just boiled, but is off the boil. Use as pure a water as possible, bottled if you can. Be aware that very hard water can prevent plants fully releasing their active principles. Allow the herb to steep for 10 minutes, then strain and store for up to 48 hours. Keep covered and in a cool place while storing.

DOSAGE: 1 TEACUP (200ML/7FL OZ) 3 TIMES A DAY FOR ADULTS.
          HALF DOSE FOR CHILDREN OR THE VERY ELDERLY.

Decoction

This is a more vigorous way of extracting herbal properties, which is used when plant parts are tougher. In a saucepan, place 300g (10½oz) of dried herb or 600g (21oz) of fresh herbs in 750ml (26 fl oz) of cold water. Make sure the plant parts are bruised and crushed for easy extraction. Heat the water to boiling point and then simmer until the liquid is reduced by about a quarter, which will take somewhere between ten minutes and half and hour. Strain, preferably through muslin, as the liquid may be 'bitty', and store, as for infusions.

DOSAGE: 1 TEACUP (200ML/7FL OZ) 3 TIMES A DAY FOR ADULTS.
            HALF DOSE FOR CHILDREN OR THE VERY ELDERLY.

Tinctures

Tinctures are also a very good way of preparing medicinal herbs, with the main benefit being that you can make up a batch which will store for a long period, saving the need to make fresh supplies every few days. Tinctures should be made from fresh herbs, preferably. Put 225g (8oz) of fresh herbs or 110g (4oz) of dried herbs in a container with a tight lid, not metal or plastic, preferably glass. Add 570ml (20 fl oz) of liquid (50% alcohol/50% pure water). The alcohol needs to be at least 40% volume – either brandy or vodka is ideal. Stand the mixture in a warm place for two weeks then strain through muslin and store in a dark glass bottle, where it can be kept for at least 12 months.

DOSAGE: 5ML 3 TIMES A DAY FOR ADULTS
            HALF DOSAGE FOR CHILDREN OR THE VERY ELDERLY

You may find that adding a little honey to the tincture makes it more palatable.

Pills, powders and ointments

You can prepare these yourself but they are very time consuming. It is also difficult to obtain accurate dosages within the confines of a private home – in other words it is not just the amount of herb you have to calculate, but making sure you have captured the essential properties of the plant is far from easy. Far better buy these off the shelf, readymade by a professional.

Hot and cold compresses (For external use only)

Use a piece of clean cotton or linen. Soak it in a hot infusion or decoction and apply to the skin, as hot as the patient can stand. Bind it in place with clingfilm and put a towel over the top to keep in the heat. This procedure can be repeated several times as the bandage cools. For a cold compress, simply allow the cloth to cool before applying.

Poultice (*For external use only*)

A poultice is the same as a compress, except that actual plant parts are placed on the body rather than a cloth soaked in extracted liquid. Mash the herb and either heat it by mixing it with a little boiled water, or heat over a pan of boiling water. Apply directly to the skin, as hot as you can bear it, and bind in place with gauze. If you have to use dried herbs, rather than fresh, for your poultice, make the dried herb into a paste and then lay it on top of some gauze with another piece of gauze on top. In other words, create a sort of sandwich. Do not put dried herbs directly onto the skin as they may irritate.

Herbal medicines are often very effective for children. Offer half the recommended dose to children under twelve.

Herbal medicines work very well for animals. To establish the correct dosage, assume the average adult weighs 9 stone (57kg). Weigh your pet and calculate on that basis.

If you are pregnant, I strongly advise you to take only absolutely essential medication. The only herbs I recommend in pregnancy are ginger root and raspberry leaf, both of which are safe and very effective.

Most herbs can be safely taken with other herb products. However, if you wish to mix prescription and herbal medicines, it is best to seek advice before doing so. Particularly avoid taking a prescription and herbal medicine for the same complaint.

AGNUS CASTUS

The most distinctive feature of agnus castus is that it has a hormonal effect on the body, significantly increasing the progesterone levels in women. This is very helpful for women suffering from PMS and particularly menopausal symptoms. Agnus castus will ease problems during periods, such as breast swelling and tenderness, bloating, irritability and depression. It also promotes regular periods and reduces the instances of acne and migraine when these symptoms are linked to the menstrual cycle.

However, agnus castus is gaining an increasing reputation as an effective alternative to HRT, relieving many of the distressing symptoms associated with the menopause. It is very important that agnus castus is not taken alongside HRT; it is a substitute for it and must be taken as an alternative. We have literally hundreds of customers who are regularly taking agnus castus during the menopause, including the author (!) and I have to say we find it an excellent alternative to HRT.

Agnus castus is also very helpful in aiding conception when infertility is due to low progesterone levels. It is important to remember this when taking agnus castus, as it is likely to increase fertility.

Although generally it is recommended that agnus castus be taken twice a day, I would recommend that your dosage should be taken in total on waking in the morning, as this has proved to be most effective.

Combinations
AGNUS CASTUS with BLACK COHOSH for menopausal and pre-menstrual problems.
AGNUS CASTUS, BLACK COHOSH and SAGE for menopausal problems where hot flushes are a feature.
AGNUS CASTUS with FEVERFEW for menstrual migraines.
AGNUS CASTUS with ECHINACEA ROOT for acne with a hormonal cause – particularly helpful for teenage girls.

AGRIMONY

Agrimony is a very helpful herb for weak stomachs. This includes indigestion, an acid stomach, a sluggish liver, general debility and gall bladder disorders. Agrimony is also very useful in the prevention of bedwetting and incontinence and eases diarrhoea. It is a particularly helpful herb for treating children.

Agrimony is a diuretic and has a long tradition for use as a spring tonic to cleanse the whole digestive system. It is the astringent activity of the herb which makes it particularly valuable for cleansing and toning the digestive tract. Agrimony is also used in the treatment of cystitis.

Agrimony is also helpful when made up into a gargle for sore throats and laryngitis, and in ancient times was used to cleanse sores and wounds.

However, it is for stomach problems that agrimony is best known, and is a very useful herb to keep in the house for this reason.

Combinations

AGRIMONY with CORIANDER to ease diarrhoea in children, as well as adults.
AGRIMONY with HORSETAIL for urinary incontinence.

ALOE VERA

Aloe vera is to be found in many tropical regions, but it is native to Africa. Cleopatra is said to have attributed her legendary beauty to the plant and certainly aloe vera gel is wonderful for the skin. The clear sap from the leaves has marvellous healing qualities for burns, wounds or any inflammation of the skin. Armies across the globe in ancient times would carry a cart into battle, containing a large aloe vera plant, so that the fresh leaves could be broken off to tend the wounded.

Aloe vera is also very helpful when used externally for sunburn, in order to reduce scarring, and indeed was made famous in modern times for its use in the healing of radiation burns. Aloe vera is also helpful for acne, varicose veins and ulcers.

Taken internally, aloe vera eases gastritis and peptic ulcers. It is often used as a general tonic to promote well-being, particularly of the gut, having gained a reputation for being helpful in the treatment of irritable bowel syndrome and ulcerated colitis. Low doses of aloe vera stimulate the digestion, higher doses act as a laxative and purgative.

While we may only be able to aspire to Cleopatra's beauty, aloe vera does improve how we look, both outside and inside!

Combinations

ALOE VERA used externally with MARIGOLD or CALENDULA for inflamed skin.
ALOE VERA taken internally with GERANIUM and PEPPERMINT for irritable bowel syndrome.

ARNICA

I always describe arnica ointment as an absolute must for the mothers of sons! This is the ideal treatment for bruises sustained in falls from bikes or in the thick of a rugby scrum. Arnica should not be applied to broken skin. It is for bruising, sprains and general aches and pains. For this reason, as well as for sporty boys, arnica is very helpful in the treatment of neuralgia and for rubbing on rheumatic joints. It is also very good when severe bruising occurs after surgical operations. With operations in mind, take homeopathic arnica internally for a week or two before a planned operation and you should find that this will help greatly reduce the discomfort of bruising and swelling which so often accompanies even quite minor surgery. Always consult your surgeon first about the use of herbal or homeopathic medicines though.

Arnica has a justifiable reputation for relieving the symptoms of shock. Following shock, homeopathic arnica should be taken every thirty minutes until the patient feels calmer.

What is not so well known, is that arnica helps restore hair loss by stimulating the blood circulation. Apply cream or diluted tincture to the affected areas and support with a vitamin B supplement.

Combinations
ARNICA diluted with WITCH HAZEL for broken or lacerated skin.
ARNICA ointment with VITAMIN B for hair loss.

ARTICHOKE

Globe artichokes are a wonderful liver restorative. Artichoke helps with the flow of bile and the digestion of fats. Take for gall bladder disorders and also liver damage, whether that be due to hepatitis, cirrhosis or liver enlargement. A liver under stress responds very well to artichoke.

Artichoke also stimulates the metabolism, aids release of fluid retention and is a general detoxifier. Artichoke also helps relieve nausea and is a general diuretic. If you are taking artichoke in the form of tincture, capsules or powders take them morning or evening before meals so that the artichoke is already in place to support the digestion. Alternatively, fresh globe artichoke can be eaten as a vegetable.

Increasingly it is being recognised that a malfunctioning liver is often at the root of many of today's ailments. Obesity on the one hand, a poor appetite and lethargy on the other, may all be caused by a liver under stress. We eat far too much fat in our modern diet and artichoke aids the breakdown and digestion of fats. Headaches, depression, lack of energy may all be improved by a stimulated liver.

Combinations
ARTICHOKE with MILK THISTLE and DANDELION for cirrhosis of the liver, particularly where alcohol is the main contributor.

BARBERRY BARK

Barberry is best known as a liver stimulant. It is helpful in the treatment of a sluggish liver, jaundice and also acts as a tonic for both the spleen and the pancreas, actually helping to reduce an enlarged spleen. Barberry is also known for its properties as a digestive tonic, easing symptoms of biliousness, gastritis and diarrhoea. It is an important antiseptic and anti-inflammatory herb and is helpful with minor infections such as mouth ulcers and more serious infections such as toxaemia from drugs or environmental chemicals.

Barberry is a mild laxative and is particularly useful in the treatment of weak or debilitated people, after perhaps a long illness. Barberry strengthens and cleanses the system, gently.

It is also known to ease bladder disorders and renal colic, and is widely used in the treatment of shingles and gallstones. It has also been used for many years in the treatment of malaria. A very diverse herb but probably at its best in the treatment of the liver.

Combinations
BARBERRY with DANDELION and ARTICHOKE for liver disorders.
BARBERRY with YARROW for malaria.
BARBERRY with FRINGE TREE bark for skin disorders.

BLACK COHOSH

This plant originates from North America where it is known as 'Squawroot' and much prized by the Native Americans. This is a very valuable herb, especially for women. It helps to relieve menstrual cramps and pains, indeed all menstrual problems where oestrogen production is low. It is particularly useful during the menopause, relieving hot flushes, general debility and depression. It is best taken with agnus castus during the menopause for maximum benefit and, together, they form a natural alternative to HRT, with a growing reputation for the treatment of menopausal symptoms. There have been a number of clinical trials, mostly in Germany, which have indicated the value of black cohosh, especially in reducing hot flushes.

Black cohosh is also extremely useful for the treatment of rheumatic problems, including rheumatoid arthritis and inflammatory arthritis – especially when these are associated with the menopause. Black cohosh is also helpful in the easing of headaches and is starting to be used in the treatment of osteoporosis. It is also of great value in lowering high blood pressure and, when combined with ginkgo, is very effective in the treatment of tinnitus.

Black cohosh is used in Chinese herbal medicine for the treatment of asthma, headaches and the relief of toxicity.

Combinations
BLACK COHOSH with AGNUS CASTUS for the menopause.
BLACK COHOSH with GINKGO LEAF for tinnitus.
BLACK COHOSH, WILD YAM and DEVIL'S CLAW for rheumatism and arthritis, particularly associated with the menopause.
BLACK COHOSH with ST JOHN'S WORT for hot flushing in the menopause, particularly where depression is also a feature.

BLUE FLAG

Blue flag is used primarily as a remedy for ailments of the liver, urinary and glandular systems. Full doses of blue flag will produce prompt and rapid bowel evacuation which can be debilitating if you are in a weakened state – so take care with the use of this herb. Blue flag is anti-inflammatory, astringent, a diuretic, a laxative and a blood and lymph purifier. It is also anti-obesity, and helps reduce liver stagnation.

Indeed, blue flag generally improves the sluggish workings of the liver and the gall bladder, whose poor performance often leads to chronic skin conditions such as acne, psoriasis and herpes. Blue flag is helpful in the treatment of cirrhosis and also hepatitis, jaundice and chronic rheumatism.

Blue flag is generally very effective in reducing a craving for food, probably because the body is kept so active eliminating it!

Combinations
BLUE FLAG and MILK THISTLE for chronic liver conditions such as cirrhosis.
BLUE FLAG and YELLOW DOCK for lymph cleansing.
BLUE FLAG and FEVERFEW for migraine and sick headaches, particularly of liver origin.

BUCHU LEAF

Buchu leaf has a distinct aroma of blackcurrants and is a native plant to South Africa. It is best known as a urinary antiseptic, which makes it particularly helpful for cystitis, thrush and problems of the prostrate. It acts as a diuretic and has a stimulating effect on the kidneys; indeed it is one of the best and most useful herbs in urinary tract diseases. Buchu's healing and soothing powers make it especially helpful to painful and burning urination.

Buchu leaf also helps reduce the effects of wind and bloating which prompts my children to refer to it as the 'anti-fart herb', which indeed it is!

Buchu leaf was first exported to Britain in 1790 and in 1821 became an official medicine, being listed 'as a remedy for cystitis, urethritis and catarrh of the bladder'.

Combinations

BUCHU LEAF with DAMIANA for cystitis.
BUCHU LEAF with WILLOW BARK for prostatitis.
BUCHU LEAF with MARSHMALLOW for irritable bladder.

BURDOCK ROOT

Burdock root is a native of both Europe and Asia, thriving in meadows and roadsides. In China it is cultivated and it is the root of this plant, which is the useful part. In both Western and Chinese medicine burdock root has traditionally been used for detoxification, where infection and fever is present such as in tonsillitis, mumps and measles.

However, burdock root is probably best known, and is most useful, in treating serious skin disorders of all kinds – acne, boils, abscesses and localised skin infections. More recently it has acquired a growing reputation for the treatment of both eczema and psoriasis. It is a herb, which is rarely used on its own and is mostly combined with others for maximum activity. It is believed that the action of burdock root is to draw toxins out of the cells into the intestinal fluid and from there into the blood stream. It is important, therefore, not to give too high a dosage of burdock root as otherwise it will create a rapid increase in toxins in the blood stream which, in turn, will have the effect of actually aggravating skin problems. It is therefore best to start with a low dosage and slowly increase.

It is also believed that burdock is helpful in aiding detoxification in cancer.

Combinations
BURDOCK ROOT with DANDELION, ECHINACEA or MARIGOLD for skin problems such as acne and boils.
BURDOCK ROOT with MARIGOLD and ECHINACEA for chronic infections such as tonsillitis.
BURDOCK ROOT with ECHINACEA, THYME and GOLDEN SEAL for candidiasis.
BURDOCK ROOT with RED CLOVER for psoriasis.

CELERY SEED

Celery seed was used in China in the 5th century BC. It was also a favourite of the pharaohs in Egypt. The plant as a whole was used as a food, and as a medicine, but it is the seeds, which are probably best known for their medicinal properties today.

Celery seed eases the pain and inflammation of arthritic and rheumatic conditions, and is particularly useful in rheumatoid arthritis where there is associated mental depression. It is also helpful in 'hot' arthritic conditions such as osteoarthritis. Gout sufferers find that regular use of celery seed greatly decreases their symptoms.

Celery seed also acts as a diuretic, stimulates detoxification via the kidneys and disinfects the bladder and urinary tubes.

Celery seed is helpful for chest problems such as asthma, bronchitis and aids the lowering of blood pressure, It is also a mild sedative.

Combinations
CELERY SEED with HAWTHORN BERRY for asthma and bronchitis.
CELERY SEED with WILLOW BARK and DANDELION for gout and arthritis.
CELERY SEED with BUCHU LEAF for cystitis.

CHAMOMILE FLOWERS

Chamomile is one of the most useful herbs. It is so calming and a mild sedative but in addition, it helps make the body receptive to other herbal medicines. In other words, it opens the gates to healing! As well as aiding sleep, chamomile flowers are anti-inflammatory and ease gastro intestinal upsets and ulcers. Chamomile flowers also help irritable bowel syndrome and colitis, as well as combating insomnia, and easing the anxiety and stress, which often accompanies the inability to sleep.

Chamomile flowers also help with digestive cramps, discomfort and acidic indigestion, pre-menstrual tension and period cramps. So many pains of the digestive system can be caused by nervousness, tension and stress and this is where chamomile is really helpful.

For external use chamomile is a wonderful ointment for the very young, the very old and for anybody with a fine sensitive skin. It is a very good natural product for nappy rash and also sore nipples during breast-feeding.

Combinations
CHAMOMILE can be used with almost any herb to calm the body and make it more receptive to the benefits of herbal medicine. However it is particularly valuable as follows:
CHAMOMILE FLOWERS with VALERIAN ROOT for gastric problems.
CHAMOMILE FLOWERS with PEPPERMINT for dyspepsia.
CHAMOMILE FLOWERS with CRANESBILL for inflammation of the upper digestive tracts.

CHICKWEED

Chickweed grows in every corner of the globe to the consternation of gardeners and farmers alike. However, before grubbing it out of your garden, it is worthwhile considering this plant's wonderful properties!

For thousands of years chickweed was used as a vegetable and still is today in China, where it is considered a delicacy. The plant grows on straggly brittle stems but the oval leaves are succulent and contain both vitamin C and phosphorous. Because of these properties, in Eastern Europe, chickweed is given to malnourished children as a tonic.

However, it is as an ointment that chickweed has really come into its own in the last few years. Eczema has always been around but today, with the amount of pollutants in the atmosphere, the skin complaint has become almost an epidemic, particularly among children. It appears that children's skin is becoming allergic to the environment. Chickweed ointment is wonderfully effective for eczema and can be used on the most delicate baby skin. It soothes and heals rapidly with no side effects. So often the frequent use of a cream sets up its own reaction on the skin being treated, but not so with chickweed. It can be used as frequently as you like. Chickweed ointment is helpful to any dry, flaky or irritated skin and relieves inflammation in sores or ulcers, helps draw splinters and stings and promotes the healing of minor burns or scalds. It is also helpful in the treatment of psoriasis.

Although not one of the major herbs for rheumatism, chickweed in tincture form, is used in the treatment of rheumatism and a pad soaked in a hot diluted tincture eases pain when placed on rheumatic joints.

Combinations

CHICKWEED ointment applied externally, and GINSENG taken internally, are a good combination in the treatment of psoriasis if the condition is largely stress-related.

CHICKWEED ointment applied externally, and ECHINACEA taken internally, will ease psoriasis if the root cause for flare-ups is a lowered immune system.

CINNAMON BARK

I always consider cinnamon bark most useful as a remedy for colds and flu, although cinnamon does have many other uses. Certainly an infusion of bark made into a hot tea with a dash of honey is really helpful in the treatment of colds and flu. However, cinnamon bark is also used as an anti-spasmodic antiseptic. It is believed to stimulate bone healing and is anti-diabetic.

Cinnamon is also particularly useful for the weak digestion, a feeble appetite, easing symptoms of diarrhoea, flatulence and vomiting. Its hyper acidity promotes the secretion of gastric juices and it is also helpful in the treatment of irritable bowel syndrome.

Combinations
CINNAMON BARK with CHAMOMILE for stomach upsets.
CINNAMON BARK with ELDERFLOWERS and PEPPERMINT for influenza.

COMFREY

A hundred years ago no self-respecting housewife would have been without a pot of comfrey in her first aid box. Cuts, bruises, fractures, sprains, acne, boils, joint pain ... are all helped by comfrey.

The herb contains allantoin which encourages the growth of bone cartilage and muscle cells. Obviously these days, any major fractures are dealt with in hospital, but breaks to fingers and toes are often untreatable and doctors simply leave them to sort themselves out. In this instance, the use of comfrey can be invaluable. So all the minor bumps and bruises of every day life could not be better treated than with comfrey which will reduce swelling and aid fast healing to minimise scars.

Comfrey is also said to be helpful for rheumatoid arthritis if used externally as a massage cream.

Taken internally, comfrey has a reputation for healing any form of laceration in the intestinal tract. It is helpful for colitis and hiatus hernias. Any form of internal bleeding benefits from comfrey as it greatly reduces blood clotting time. For this reason it was once used extensively in the treatment of tuberculosis and pleurisy.

Combinations
COMFREY with MARSH MALLOW and MEADOWSWEET for gastric ulcers and inflammations.
COMFREY with COLTSFOOT and WHITE HOREHOUND for chest and bronchial problems.

CORNSILK

Cornsilk has a beneficial and soothing effect on the kidneys. The herb is traditionally considered to be very effective in reducing kidney stone formation and relieving some of the symptoms associated with existing kidney stones. It also appears to have a soothing and relaxing effect on the lining of the urinary tubes and bladder, improving urine flow and relieving irritation. It is, therefore, very effective in the treatment of chronic cystitis, irritation of the bladder and, indeed, any situation where the passing of urine is difficult – ie prostate enlargement.

Cornsilk is also thought to improve the flow of bile through the bile duct, and in China it has a reputation for improving blood pressure and avoiding the formation of blood clots.

Cornsilk is often thought to be at its most effective taken as an infusion.

Cornmeal mashed up and made into a hot poultice is very much a part of American folk medicine for the treatment of bruises, sores and boils. It is understood that Native Americans rarely suffered from kidney or bladder problems due to the amount of corn in their diet.

Combinations
CORNSILK with ECHINACEA and BUCHU for chronic cystitis.
CORNSILK with ECHINACEA and PARSLEY PIERT for kidney stones.

COUCHGRASS

This is the grass to which dogs go when sick, if they can, and like much instinctive animal behaviour, we can learn a thing or two from them. Couchgrass acts as a diuretic and soothes inflammation of the urinary tract. It is a urinary antiseptic and is also a laxative It is a useful anti-cholesterol.

Couchgrass is frequently used in the treatment of cystitis, urethritis, liver disorder, renal colic and kidney stones. It is of value in the treatment of enlarged prostate glands.

It is also useful in the treatment of gout and rheumatism and particularly backache, easing painful inflammation.

Couchgrass also eases the symptoms of chronic skin disease.

Couchgrass is best taken as a herbal tea – three cups of tea a day after meals.

Combinations

COUCHGRASS with HYDRANGEA for prostatitis.
COUCHGRASS with BUCHU and YARROW for cystitis and urethritis.

CRAMP BARK

Cramp bark is the number one herb for muscular spasms and cramp. It deals with any form of muscle tension which causes prolonged pain or continual aching.

Cramp bark is extensively used for menstrual and ovarian cramp (period pains). It is best taken several days before menstruation and then during the length of the period. It is also very helpful for the aches and pains of the menopause.

Cramp bark can be taken for any condition where muscle relaxation is required or where muscular tension exists. It can be taken after exercise or injury and because this useful herb has mildly sedative constituents, it makes it all the more effective in dealing with pain.

Cramp bark is also anti-spasmpodic and improves blood flow. It is therefore used in the treatment of such wide-ranging conditions as high blood pressure, osteoartritis, angina and irritable bowel syndrome.

Cramp bark has some astringent action which is why it is often associated with curing infantile bed wetting and general incontinence.

With our damp climate, it is said that at least half the population of the United Kingdom suffers from back pain at some point in their lives, so it is well worth mentioning that cramp bark is especially helpful in the treatment of back pain.

Combinations
CRAMP BARK with CRANESBILL for incontinence.
CRAMP BARK with WILLOW BARK for pain.
CRAMP BARK with AGNUS CASTUS for menstrual pain.
CRAMP BARK with ST JOHN'S WORT for back ache.
CRAMP BARK with CHAMOMILE and VALERIAN for irritable bowel syndrome.

DAMIANA

Damiana herb is native to the Gulf of Mexico and Southern California. It also grows in the Northern Caribbean islands, preferring a hot humid climate.

While damiana has a reputation for easing many problems, it is probably best known for its aphrodisiac qualities. Though seen principally as aiding male problems – impotence and premature ejaculation – it is also very beneficial for women, restoring and stimulating the reproductive organs of both sexes. Damiana is also useful for painful and delayed periods, and quite specifically, for menstrual headaches.

Damiana is also considered an excellent tonic for the nervous system and is said to have a life-enhancing and stimulating effect on mind and body. Damiana is often given for mild to moderate depression and nervous exhaustion and is a very good treatment for on-going anxiety and stress, particularly where stress has been present for a long time.

Damiana is also useful in the treatment of urinary infections, being a urinary antiseptic, diuretic and mild laxative.

Combinations

DAMIANA with ST JOHN'S WORT for depression.
DAMIANA with FEVERFEW for menstrual migraine.
DAMIANA with KOREAN GINSENG for sexual dysfunction.

DANDELION LEAF

Dandelion leaf grows almost throughout the world and when the leaves are young they are often used as a vegetable.

As a herbal medicine dandelion is one of the most commonly used detoxifying herbs. Working on the liver, gall bladder and kidneys, it stimulates the removal of waste via the bowel and in urine. Conventional diuretics lead to a loss of potassium in the body but dandelion contains such high levels of potassium itself, that the body loses none of this important mineral. Dandelion is a particularly valuable herb for the liver and has a significant detoxifying effect upon it.

Dandelion is also of great value in arthritic conditions such as osteoarthritis and gout. It is also very helpful where fluid retention is a problem – in the case of swollen ankles or bloated abdomen and premenstrual fluid retention.

Dandelion is marvellous for warts. Apply the white juice that comes from both stem and leaves twice a day for a few weeks and you will be amazed by the results.

Combinations
DANDELION with CELERY SEED and WILLOW BARK for gout and osteoarthritis.
DANDELION with HAWTHORN BERRY and GARLIC for high blood pressure.
DANDELION with MILK THISTLE for liver repair.

DEVIL'S CLAW

This herb is best known for easing arthritis and rheumatism, particularly where pain is the main feature. It has been compared with cortisone in terms of effect. For best results devil's claw does need to be taken over a number of weeks and it is particularly good for persistent back pain. It is a very useful anti-inflammatory herb and for that reason is often very effective in the treatment of inflamed joints. Devil's claw is helpful in the treatment of gout, osteoarthritis, fibrositis and rheumatoid arthritis, and reduces fevers.

Devil's claw is also helpful for a poor digestive system, it helps to stimulate activity while at the same time bringing soothing relief. Devil's claw is also useful for liver and gall bladder complaints.

Used externally devil's claw is excellent for the treatment of sores, ulcers and boils.

Devil's claw is also hyper-tensive and decreases the heart rate.

Combinations

DEVIL'S CLAW with BLACK COHOSH and ST JOHN'S WORT for rheumatoid arthritis.
DEVIL'S CLAW with WILLOW BARK for osteoarthritis.
DEVIL'S CLAW with ANGELICA to cleanse the digestive system.

ECHINACEA ROOT

I believe echinacea is one of the most important medicinal herbs because it boosts the immune system – in other words it helps the body to help itself. Antibiotics have their place and in many cases are life saving, but over recent years the Western World has been subject to antibiotic abuse and the result has been the lowering of our natural resistance, allowing for the growth of so called super bugs. Echinacea is a safe and effective alternative.

Echinacea root is anti-viral and anti-bacterial. It helps combat minor infections such as coughs and colds but it is also very effective in fighting chronic infections such as ME. By taking echinacea root in advance of infection, one greatly reduces the chance of developing flu, colds and respiratory tract infections. It is also very helpful with throat problems such as tonsillitis and quinsy. How many times have you been told 'It's just a virus, there is no treatment'? Echinacea will arm your body to fight off viruses.

Echinacea root is also very helpful in combating skin infections such as acne, boils and even psoriasis. Echinacea root will treat any infection where the underlying toxicity within the body is likely to be the cause of the problem – ie an infected cut or a tooth abscess will respond well to echinacea root. This is a truly wonderful herb.

Combinations
ECHINACEA with GARLIC for throat infections.
ECHINACEA with SAGE and GINGER ROOT for gastroenteritis.
ECHINACEA with ST JOHN'S WORT and/or LEMON BALM for viral infections.
ECHINACEA with CHICKWEED ointment for psoriasis.
ECHINACEA with GOLDEN SEAL for conjunctivitis.
ECHINACEA with AGNUS CASTUS for acne with an hormonal cause ie particularly helpful for teenage girls.
ECHINACEA with MARIGOLD ointment for chronic skin conditions.

ELDERFLOWER

Elderflower is an excellent home treatment for everyday coughs, cold and flu. Elderflower helps balance circulation and therefore has a cooling effect and helps lower fever. The flowers also tone up the mucus membranes of both the nose and the throat and generally Elderflower improves resistance to infection.

Elderflower is also helpful in the release of irritations and allergies which makes it useful in the treatment of hayfever. An infusion of elderflower should be taken three times a day up to three months before the hayfever season to help reduce attacks. Elderflower is not a 'cure all' for hayfever. It may still be necessary to take some other medication as well for severe attacks, but certainly it is likely to reduce the symptoms and in the case of children maybe enough on its own. Elderflower is helpful in the treatment of chronic catarrh and is also a very useful remedy for ear infections.

Over many centuries elderflower water has been used to whiten the skin and remove freckles. Elder leaves are excellent for chilblains and bruising.

The berries of elderflower are rich in vitamin C and have been used traditionally for rheumatism and are helpful in improving eyesight. They are also considered to be a mild laxative.

Combinations
ELDERFLOWER with YARROW and PEPPERMINT for fevers and influenza type infections.
ELDERFLOWER with NETTLE for hayfever.
ELDERFLOWER with ECHINACEA for ear infections.

EUCALYPTUS

Eucalyptus, to this day, is widely used by the Aborigines of Australia They consider it to be a kind of 'cure all'. Eucalyptus is antibiotic, anti-viral, anti-fungal and anti-spasmodic. It is prized for its general restorative features and has a reputation for dealing with a wide variety of feverish complaints – no wonder the Aborigines value it so highly!

More specifically, eucalyptus reduces fevers, helps with asthma and nasal catarrh, bronchitis, sinusitis, sore throats and any respiratory disorders. It is best used, in these circumstances, either as an inhalant or as a chest rub.

Traditionally eucalyptus was used in the treatment of diphtheria and tuberculosis when both diseases were common in this country.

Eucalyptus is also helpful in the treatment of headaches brought on by congestion and fever.

In some parts of the world, eucalyptus leaves are smoked for relief from asthma and the Chinese use a few drops of eucalyptus oil in water as a cleansing douse in the case of a variety of sexually transmitted diseases.

Combinations
EUCALYPTUS is generally used as a treatment on its own but it should not be given with GOLDEN SEAL, with which it is antagonistic.
EUCALYPTUS OIL – a few drops of oil in wine is said to heal infected cuts.

FENNEL

Fennel is a gentle warming herb ideal for delicate stomachs and mild digestive problems. Fennel tea is often given to colicky babies and does prove very helpful, not only in easing the pain of the colic but also arousing the appetite. It is also a helpful anti-spasmodic in young children.

Fennel soothes irritable bowels. It is anti-inflammatory, it aids digestion, it is a diuretic and in all cases, the action is very mild and gentle. For this reason, fennel is suitable for the very old as well as the very young, or indeed anyone who is of a particularly delicate disposition, perhaps after serious illness.

Fennel is good to take as a tea during lactation in that it helps increase milk in the nursing mother.

Fennel tea is also very helpful in the treatment of obesity, to be drunk instead of traditional tea and coffee.

It is generally believed that fennel tea will smooth wrinkles if taken internally. This property appears in many of the old herb books I have studied and I can only assume that because of the gentle nature of fennel, it stops one frowning, hence smoothing out the wrinkles! Well, anything is worth a try!

Fennel is often used externally as an eyewash and is very helpful for red and tired eyes.

Combinations
FENNEL tea is good to take alongside any herbal medicine you select for the treatment of the digestive system.

FENUGREEK

Fenugreek is one of the oldest medicinal herbs. It was used in ancient Egypt to ease the pain of childbirth and even today Egyptian women will take it for period pain. Today, fenugreek is best known as a 'tummy herb'. Most minor problems of the intestine, bowels and stomach are greatly helped by fenugreek. This includes irritable bowel, colitis, stomach ulcers, inflammation, diarrhoea and gastro-enteritis. It is helpful in the treatment of Crohn's disease and also where the patient has a weak digestion, poor appetite and general debility. It is also taken where the patient has cancer of the bowel as it is both soothing and mildly analgesic.

Fenugreek is good in the treatment of sore gums and mouth ulcers, also chronic coughs and bronchitis. Fenugreek is used in Chinese medicine for kidney complaints and protection against thrombosis, embolism and angina.

The seeds of fenugreek are traditionally used as an aphrodisiac, having a reputation for the treatment of male impotence.

Fenugreek is a safe and soothing herb which combines well with others to enhance its efficiency.

Combinations

FENUGREEK and GOLDEN SEAL for stomach and intestinal problems.
FENUGREEK with WILD YAM for diverticulitis.
FENUGREEK with SLIPPERY ELM for mouth ulcers.
FENUGREEK with CRANESBILL for diarrhoea.

FEVERFEW

Clinical trials in the mid 1980s established feverfew as the migraine herb. Certainly it is very effective for migraine sufferers, although it has little effect once the migraine has really established itself. Ideally you should take small doses of feverfew as a preventative treatment, increasing the dose as you feel the migraine coming on. Being able to predict the onset of a migraine greatly enhances the value of feverfew. For example, if you have a migraine associated with the menstrual cycle, then regulating a preventative dose is relatively easy. For others it is not so easy – you could have migraine associated with stress, overwork, emotional upsets, lack of sleep – even bright lights can bring it on – in these cases it is more difficult to predict. If this is your problem, take feverfew in any circumstance where you feel that it is likely a migraine might develop – it will do you no harm and there are no side effects.

Feverfew is also excellent for ordinary headache sufferers and has long been recognised as a splendid cure for hangovers! It is also very helpful for both arthritic and rheumatic pain particularly if either are inflammatory.

Feverfew also has a reputation for protection against clot formation. This makes it a particularly useful herb to take on long flights as not only will it help reduce the chances of deep vein thrombosis but will treat the headaches often associated with travel.

If you decide to use fresh feverfew leaves instead of capsules, be aware that they are absolutely disgusting to eat and may give you mouth ulcers if you do not gargle thoroughly when you have forced them down!

Combinations

FEVERFEW with WILLOW BARK for inflammatory joint pain.
FEVERFEW with AGNUS CASTUS for menstrual migraines.
FEVERFEW with DAMIANA for migraine linked with nervous exhaustion.

GARLIC

Garlic has been around for at least five thousand years. As a prized medicine, it has long been known to reduce blood cholesterol levels and hence reduce the risk of heart attacks. Even traditional medicine recognises the value of garlic for heart patients to help lower the risk of further heart attacks. Garlic is also an excellent remedy for chesty conditions and bronchitis, actually reducing infection which may develop in lungs or airways. It is also very important for circulation and increases blood thinning, thus helping protect against strokes. Garlic is also excellent when used in the treatment of raised cholesterol levels.

It is a well-established fact that the pyramids were built on garlic – it was given to the labourers in large quantities to keep them fit and healthy during their long and difficult work. That was in about 4500 BC!

Before penicillin and antibiotics, garlic was usually one of the first treatments given to fight against any form of infection. It was used to dress wounds in the trenches during the First World War – it is an excellent antiseptic dressing. Also when used externally, garlic cream is anti-fungal and therefore marvellous for athlete's foot, rashes and warts.

Combinations

GARLIC with HAWTHORN BERRY and DANDELION LEAF for high blood pressure.
GARLIC with GINGER ROOT for digestive infections.
GARLIC with ECHINACEA ROOT for viral and chronic infections, particularly of the throat and chest.

GENTIAN

Gentian is an Alpine herb which is grown in mountainous regions right across central and southern Europe. It is the root which is the valuable part of the plant. Gentian is used primarily in the treatment of a weak digestion and under activity, particularly of the stomach. Gentian stimulates the digestive juices and accelerates the emptying of the stomach. Gentian also aids in the absorption of nutrients and will ease the side effects of poor digestion – ie wind, indigestion, poor appetite, and stimulates the production of saliva. Gentian is frequently used when a patient fails to gain weight, perhaps after illness.

The fact that gentian helps in the absorption of nutrients is important, as it is very helpful in the treatment of anaemic patients where there is an iron deficiency. For this reason gentian is often given in small quantities for people suffering from heavy menstrual bleeding.

As well as stimulating the digestion gentian also stimulates liver and gall bladder activity.

Combinations
GENTIAN with GINGER to stimulate appetite.

GINGER ROOT

Ginger root is highly effective for preventing travel sickness and general nausea. It works by calming the gastro-intestinal tract. It is also an antiseptic and therefore can be used for gut infections due to food poisoning and dysentery. It can be safely used for morning sickness, and half doses are ideal for children who suffer from car sickness. It is also helpful for baby colic.

Ginger root is also very useful for easing the symptoms of coughs, colds, flu and bronchitis. It is very helpful for whooping cough and by encouraging sweating, aids the lowering of body temperature during a fever. Ginger is an anti-oxidant and its anti-blood clotting properties assist in preventing strokes and improving circulation.

The warming effect of ginger when applied externally makes it very helpful for chilblains and aching muscles.

Combinations

GINGER ROOT with CHAMOMILE FLOWERS for nausea, vomiting and dyspepsia.
GINGER ROOT with GARLIC and CINNAMON for digestive infections.
GINGER ROOT with ECHINACEA ROOT for respitory infections.
GINGER ROOT with CAPSICUM for chilblains.
GINGER ROOT with GINKGO LEAF to aid stroke prevention.
GINGER ROOT with BORAGE for general bowel health.

GINKGO LEAF

Ginko is a native of China and is believed to be one of the oldest trees on the planet (at least 200 million years old). As I sit writing this book I feel deeply in need of large quantities of ginko leaf for it aids memory, concentration and improves cerebral circulation! In the 1960s, extensive research and a number of clinical trials established ginkgo as a real aid to cerebral problems and as well as concentrating the mind, it has a really useful role to play in the treatment of Alzheimer's and dementia.

In many parts of Europe, particularly France and Germany, ginkgo is taken daily by millions of people from middle age onwards to maintain and improve cerebral circulation and memory and also reduce the risk of stroke. It is also an anti-depressant and increases people's sense of well being and vitality. It is a sort of brain tonic!

Ginkgo aids in the treatment of thrombosis, tinnitus, vertigo, dizziness and any problems associated with the central nervous system which makes it helpful in the treatment of multiple sclerosis. Ginkgo helps improve circulation as a whole and therefore is useful in the treatment of heart disease.

Increasingly ginkgo is being recognised as useful in the treatment of asthma as it is anti-inflammatory and has anti-allergic activity. Ginkgo is a very important herb – particularly in the over fifties!

Combinations

GINKGO with HAWTHORN for heart disease.
GINKGO with AGNUS CASTUS for pre-menstrual tension.
GINKGO with ST JOHN'S WORT for depression, neuralgia and nervous disorders.
GINKGO with BLACK COHOSH for tinnitus.
GINKGO with GINGER to reduce the risks of strokes.
GINKGO with KOREAN GINSENG for over work and exhaustion.

GINSENG

Marco Polo described ginseng as a 'prized wonder drug'. It is a native of the Far East and has been cultivated in Korea since 1300.

Ginseng is the anti-stress herb. It eases stress both physical and mental, supporting the body to help it cope with the worst effects of fatigue and exhaustion. Yet, while it is a stimulant, if sleep is required by the exhausted body, ginseng adapts itself to act as a sedative as well. Clever stuff!

Ginseng also acts as an aphrodisiac for men and is particularly considered to be a valuable remedy for improving health and well being in old age. Traditionally, it was used during the long hard winters of Northern China to keep body and soul on an even keel. Ginseng really is an excellent treatment for people under huge strain from chronic exhaustion, long term stress and impotence and for less severe problems such as headaches, general overwork and jet lag. It is the perfect herb for today's stressful living. Marco Polo knew what he was talking about!

Combinations
GINSENG with GINKGO for overwork and exhaustion.
GINSENG with DAMIANA for male sexual dysfunction.
GINSENG with CHICKWEED OINTMENT for psoriasis.

GOLDEN SEAL

Golden seal is a native of America and was used by American Indians, particularly the Cherokees. It is considered a very potent remedy for infections of the mucus membranes throughout the whole body – ie eye, ear, throat, nose, stomach, intestines and vagina.

Golden seal is helpful in the treatment of ulcers, particularly peptic ulcers, as well as any form of infection or inflammatory problem throughout the whole gastro intestinal tract. Golden seal also stimulates bowel production and boosts the workings of both the liver and the gall bladder.

In recent times with the apparent increase in cases of psoriasis, golden seal has really come into its own in helping to reduce the severity of the skin disorder.

Golden seal taken externally can be used as an eyewash, as a mouthwash for infected gums and as a douse for the treatment of thrush and other infections.

Combinations
GOLDEN SEAL with CHAMOMILE FLOWERS for peptic ulcers and gastritis.
GOLDEN SEAL with ECHINACEA for conjunctivitis.
GOLDEN SEAL with GARLIC and GINGER ROOT for digestive infections.
GOLDEN SEAL with DANDELION for hay fever.
GOLDEN SEAL with GINSENG and CHICKWEED OINTMENT for psoriasis.

HAWTHORN BERRY

Hawthorn has flourished for centuries in the hedgerows, woods and fields throughout the British Isles and it has been well known for its medicinal properties since the sixteenth century.

While initially Hawthorn berry was used in the treatment of kidney infections and gall bladder problems, in more recent times it has been recognised as a very serious and effective heart herb. Specifically, it is used extensively in the treatment of angina and coronary artery disease. Generally it eases hypertension, aids circulation and gives cardio-vascular support.

Hawthorn is very valuable for high blood pressure sufferers and yet also helps raise low blood pressure – in other words it stabilises blood pressure at its correct level. It also assists in the stabilising of irregular heartbeats.

Hawthorn berry should be viewed as a sort of tonic food for the heart, both supporting blood flow and improving the overall heart function.

Hawthorn berry is also useful in the treatment of diarrhoea, poor digestion and bloating caused around periods and after childbirth.

Combinations
HAWTHORN BERRY with GINKGO and DANDELION LEAF for mild to moderate heart failure.
HAWTHORN BERRY with GARLIC and VALERIAN for high blood pressure.
HAWTHORN BERRY with CELERY SEED for asthma and bronchitis

HYSSOP

Hyssop is a holy herb of the ancient Greeks, prescribed by Hypocrates for pleurisy and also for asthma and catarrh. The herb's properties are anti-inflammatory and anti-viral and in today's much polluted world, it is as a relief to asthma that hyssop is becoming best known. It is also often prescribed for bronchitis and is very effective.

Hyssop is also very helpful if taken in the very early stages of cold or flu and it provides relief for digestive upsets and nervous tummies.

Hyssop helps to induce heavy sweating in fevers to bring down the body temperature. It is a mild analgesic diuretic and anti-spasmodic. The anti-spasmodic properties of hyssop make it useful in the treatment of petit mal, and also in reducing anxiety attacks and relieving hysteria.

The anti-viral property of hyssop makes it an excellent treatment for herpes, and hence cold sores.

The essential oil of the hyssop plant is uplifting to the spirits. It is particularly helpful in cases of nervous exhaustion caused by overwork and anxiety. It eases depression and reduces feelings of grief and guilt. It acts as a gentle relaxing nerve tonic which puts life back in perspective.

Combinations
HYSSOP with LIQUORICE for bronchitis.
HYSSOP with MULLEIN for stubborn coughs and weak lungs.
HYSSOP with BETONY for easing epileptic episodes.

ICELAND MOSS

Iceland moss is a very important herb and highly regarded for upper respiratory ailments. It is a useful herb for minor problems such as a dry, aggravating cough and general catarrh of the nose throat and chest. However, it is also important in the treatment of both chronic and acute bronchitis and laryngitis. Equally important, it helps arrest permanent respiratory damage by providing a protective layer to the respiratory tract, breaking up tough mucus in the respiratory organs and easing blocked sinuses.

Iceland moss is often used in wasting disease and terminal conditions where there is exhaustion and vomiting. Iceland moss improves digestion in these conditions and helps arrest the vomiting. Iceland moss is generally very helpful in treating conditions of the stomach, such as that sick feeling one gets when a cold or flu produces catarrh which often finds its way to the stomach.

In essence, therefore, iceland moss is highly active if you have any sort of chest infection and helps prevent any permanent respiratory damage.

Combinations
ICELAND MOSS and LOBELIA for catarrh.
ICELAND MOSS with LIQUORICE for bronchitis.
ICELAND MOSS with PRIMULA for productive cough.
ICELAND MOSS with SAGE for a sore throat.
ICELAND MOSS with GOLDEN SEAL for wasting disease.

LAVENDER

Lavender is a herb which tends to be associated with calm. Possibly best known for easing insomnia, lavender is also excellent for the treatment of physical and mental exhaustion. It helps to relieve stress, calms and relaxes, and is particularly helpful where the patient suffers from panic attacks.

Lavender is also an anti-depressant and anti-spasmodic. It is helpful in the treatment of depression, nervous headaches, neuralgia and rheumatism and is a general soothing tonic for the nervous system.

Lavender helps in the reduction of high blood pressure, windy colic, sinusitis and toothache! It really is a very good all rounder as herbs go, so it is small wonder lavender has been in such constant use through many centuries and was an absolute must in most English gardens. When you add to its many attributes, the pungent and oddly nostalgic scent, it proves to be a very pleasant herb to use purely for its fragrance.

Lavender oil used externally, helps prevent neuralgia, rheumatism, aching muscles and tends to introduce a feel good factor. Smear on the forehead for migraine.

Combinations
LAVENDER with LIME FLOWERS for reducing high blood pressure.
LAVENDER with VALERIAN for headaches.
LAVENDER with ROSEMARY for mild depression.

LEMON BALM

The herbalist Gerard said that Lemon balm 'comforteth the hart and driveth away all sadness'. Over the centuries, lemon balm has gathered a reputation for being the elixir of youth and certainly it is a very cheering herb. It revives and lifts the spirits, acts as a tonic, eases mild depression, restlessness and irritability. It reduces feelings of nervousness and panic and it will often calm a nervous heart, or palpations.

Lemon balm is also excellent when anxiety is interfering with normal digestion – ie a nervous tummy, causing indigestion, acidity, bloating, colic and even a peptic ulcer. Lemon balm also eases headaches, migraine and dizziness.

Used externally lemon balm is excellent for curing herpes. Applied as a cream, lotion or tincture to cold sores, not only will they tend to clear up more quickly, but also the time between outbreaks will be greatly extended. Lemon balm is good with sores generally and for painful swellings.

New research is suggesting that fresh lemon balm oil may be useful in the treatment of Alzheimer's disease.

Combinations
LEMON BALM with CHAMOMILE for digestive problems.
LEMON BALM with LIME LEAVES for palpations and panic attacks.
LEMON BALM with ECHINACEA for cold sores.
LEMON BALM with ST JOHN'S WORT and ROSEMARY for depression.

LIME FLOWERS

The chief action of lime flowers is as a sedative. They are relaxing and encourage sleep. Lime flowers are an excellent remedy for stress and panic, and for symptoms that tend to go with anxiety, such as headaches and nervous palpations. Lime flowers are also useful in the treatment of migraines and vertigo and bring relief to colds, flu and nasal catarrh.

Lime flowers are also commonly used to lower high blood pressure and here again they are particularly helpful when the high blood pressure is the result of emotional factors – ie tension, anxiety and general nervousness. However lime flowers are also used in the long term treatment of blood pressure associated with arteriosclerosis, as they aid the toning of blood vessel walls.

Lime flowers are also diuretic and mildly astringent.

Lime flowers used externally are excellent on the skin when itchy or prickly.

Combinations

LIME FLOWERS with LEMON BALM for anxiety and nervous palpations.
LIME FLOWERS with HAWTHORN for high blood pressure.
LIME FLOWERS with VALERIAN for insomnia, and high blood pressure associated with nervous tension.
LIME FLOWERS with ELDERFLOWER or ELDERBERRY for colds.

LIQUORICE

Liquorice is a very important herb, and it is the root which is the part used in herbal medicine. It is a powerful anti-inflammatory herb for the digestion and is a good treatment for respiratory problems.

Liquorice is perhaps most associated with its effect on the digestion, relieving peptic ulcers, gastritis and is particularly helpful where excessive acid is produced. However, it is also extremely helpful in many respiratory conditions such as bronchitis, asthma and dry coughs.

Liquorice is helpful with the symptoms of arthritis, particularly where the arthritis is inflamed, and with skin disorders such as psoriasis.

Liquorice is very supportive to the adrenal glands and helps in the treatment of Addision's disease, appearing to stimulate the adrenal cortex function.

Liquorice is helpful in the treatment of chronic fatigue and indeed any illness where exhaustion is a feature.

Liquorice has the ability to stimulate interferon production and therefore is useful in the treatment of hepatitis A, B and C. It is generally helpful in increasing the performance of both liver and kidneys.

Due to its oestreogenic activity, liquorice is valuable during the menopause and has been used for centuries in the treatment of hot flushes and other menopausal problems. Liquorice is useful as a gentle laxative.

Liquorice is such a helpful and useful medicinal plant, it really is a must for your herbal medicine chest!

Combinations
LIQUORICE with CHAMOMILE, GOLDEN SEAL and SLIPPERY ELM for peptic ulcers.
LIQUORICE with MILK THISTLE, ECHINACEA and GOLDEN SEAL for hepatitis.
LIQUORICE with SAGE and WILD YAM for menopausal problems.
LIQUORICE with ELECAMPANE and THYME for bronchitis and coughs.

LOBELIA

Lobelia first came to notice in the United States where it grows as a common weed. It was Samuel Thompson in the early 19th century, a renowned American herbalist, who first recognised lobelia's properties. Lobelia is a powerful anti-spasmodic and respiratory stimulant. This makes it particularly valuable in the treatment of asthma, especially bronchial asthma and also bronchitis. Lobelia works by relaxing the muscles of the small bronchial tubes therefore opening up the airways. It stimulates breathing and the coughing up of phlegm. In North America, lobelia is often combined with cayenne, the idea being that lobelia relaxes the chest and then the cayenne pepper acts as a hot stimulant to push the circulation into areas that have been opened up by the lobelia, which in turn improves blood flow.

Lobelia is also used externally very effectively for the relief of aching and tense muscles particularly in a situation where muscles have locked hard due to strain. Lobelia is also helpful with painful joints, back pain and arthritic problems.

Combinations

LOBELIA with LIQUORICE and THYME for asthma.
LOBELIA with ELECAMPANE and ECHINACEA for bronchitis.
LOBELIA with CRAMPBARK for muscle tension.
LOBELIA with VALERIAN for withdrawal from cigarette smoking addiction.

MARIGOLD

Marigold is essentially a herb for the skin, indeed it is
herbs for treating skin conditions. It is very useful
complaints, such as cuts, grazes and rashes. It is also ver
and inflamed skin, including minor burns and sunburn.   ...ps in the
treatment of acne and for fungal infections such as ringworm, athlete's
foot and thrush. Marigold is anti-inflammatory, antiseptic and anti-
fungal. It is so safe that it can be used on the most delicate skin – for
nappy rash, cradle cap, sore nipples and mastitis. No skin is too young
or too old to benefit from marigold.

However, the wonders of marigold do not end there. Taken internally, it
is excellent for inflammatory conditions of the digestive system. It is
also useful in the treatment of liver and gall bladder problems including
hepatitis. Above all, it is very effective for gastric and duodenal ulcers,
and indeed any digestive problems which could be loosely described
as indigestion.

Marigold is mildly oestreogenic and may be used for period pain and to
regulate menstrual bleeding.

Combinations
MARIGOLD with ECHINACEA ROOT and NETTLE for chronic skin
conditions and infections.
MARIGOLD with WILD YAM, AGNUS CASTUS and CRAMP BARK for
irregular and painful periods.
MARIGOLD with MARSHMALLOW ROOT and CRANESBILL for
digestive problems.

MARSHMALLOW

Marshmallow is another herb whose origins come from ancient Greece. It was much revered for its healing qualities; Hypocrates believed it was especially helpful in the treatment of wounds. Marshmallow root and leaves have been used as a vegetable through the centuries, but it is as a medicinal herb that it is best known.

Internally, marshmallow is taken for inflammation of the mucous membranes. Gastritis, enteritis, peptic ulcers and urinary infections such as cystitis, inflammation of the alimentary canal, kidneys, bladder or ulceration of the stomach and duodenum all respond to marshmallow, as does a hiatus hernia.

Marshmallow is also very good for bronchial conditions and persistent coughs and has been widely used as an expectorant. It is very helpful in the treatment of persistent catarrh. Marshmallow is very soothing for any mucous membrane irritations.

Taken externally marshmallow is excellent for wounds, burns, boils, skin ulceration and for the drawing of splinters – indeed any skin infection will respond to marshmallow.

Combinations

MARSHMALLOW with ECHINACEA ROOT for coughs and colds.
MARSHMALLOW with COMFREY and CRANESBILL for peptic ulcers.

MILK THISTLE

Milk thistle is a very attractive plant It is also a very important herbal medicine because it protects that most vital of organs – the liver. It is helpful in the treatment of hepatitis A, B and C and in any situation where the liver is under stress. This can be as a result of infection, alcohol abuse or if chemotherapy is prescribed. In the case of chemotherapy, milk thistle will help reduce potential damage to the liver and ease side effects. Milk thistle supports normal liver function and stimulates liver cell regeneration. It also has anti-oxidant action and is helpful in the treatment of bile duct problems.

Milk thistle also has a reputation for increasing breast milk production and traditionally was eaten as spring tonic, the idea being that it cleansed the whole system after the winter.

In 1597, Gerard wrote about milk thistle: 'My opinion is this is the best remedy that grows against all melancholy diseases.' Milk thistle is still today considered to be an excellent remedy for melancholia, which in itself is associated with a poor functioning liver.

Combinations
MILK THISTLE with DANDELION and ECHINACEA for hepatitis.
MILK THISTLE with DANDELION and ARTICHOKE for cirrhosis and alcohol abuse.

MINT

There are about thirty different types of mint and the properties of this wonderfully aromatic herb are endless. Wilafried of Strabo said in the 12th century: 'If any man can name all the properties of mint, he must know how many fish swim in the Indian Ocean.'

Today, peppermint tends to be the mint preferred for medicinal use in the west but garden Mint which is less strong, but just as effective, is particularly good for children. Mint is a great remedy for nausea and particularly good for travel sickness, flatulence, colic and poor appetite.

Mint generally calms the digestive tract and is a mild sedative.

Mint also helps relax muscles of the digestive tract and stimulates the bowel flow.

It is helpful both in treatment of Crohn's disease and diverticula disease.

The Chinese favour mint for head colds and influenza and also for headaches, sore throats and eye inflammations. Mint also induces sweating in fevers and therefore lowers temperatures. It is anti-bacterial and is therefore useful in combating infection.

Externally, a compress of mint infusion will cool and relieve inflamed joints, rheumatism and neuralgia. Inhale an infusion to ease nasal congestion.

Combinations
PEPPERMINT with GINGER for sickness and vomiting.

MOTHERWORT

There is an old saying which goes like this: 'Drink motherwort tea and live to be a source of continuous astonishment and frustration to waiting heirs.' This is certainly an encouraging idea!

Motherwort has a reputation for being a laxative, a diaphoretic and for generally improving the performance of the bowels. However, it is as a nerve and heart support that motherwort is probably the most effective. It is helpful in the treatment of angina and indeed any simple or uncomplicated heart condition – in other words, it is very helpful in encouraging the heart to behave normally – hence the saying about frustrating waiting heirs!

Motherwort is also very helpful in the treatment of hyperactive thyroid.

Motherwort can be taken for absent or painful menstruation, and is helpful for menopausal flushes and pre-menstrual tension. Motherwort also eases the pain of labour.

Motherwort is also said to ward off schizophrenic tendencies.

Warning – do not take during pregnancy.

Combinations
MOTHERWORT with VERVAIN for relaxing nervous conditions.
MOTHERWORT with BLACK COHOSH and CRAMP BARK for menstrual disorders.
MOTHERWORT with HAWTHORN BERRY for heart disorders.
MOTHERWORT with SKULLCAP and VALERIAN for withdrawal from benzodiazepine addiction.

MULLEIN

Mullein had a huge reputation in Ireland as the traditional treatment for tuberculosis. It was initiated by a Dr Quinlan and was known as the 'Quinlan Cure'. He maintained that the green leaves of mullein, boiled in two pints of fresh milk, then strained and sweetened with honey, soothed the lungs, increased weight and restored vitality.

The properties of mullein do support Dr Quinlan's Cure, for it is an excellent herb for soothing irritable respiratory conditions. This makes it very helpful in the treatment of asthma, deep and persistent coughs, emphysema, tracheitis and hay fever. It reduces inflammation and tones the mucous membranes.

Mullein is also used for the treatment of bed wetting.

Taken externally mullein oil is used for earache and temporary deafness. Mullein is also good for piles and pain or itching in the rectum. Mullein is very soothing and healing for wounds and ulcers.

Combinations
MULLEIN with HYSSOP for stubborn coughs and weak lungs.
MULLEIN with WHITE HOREHOUND for bronchitis.

NETTLE

Nettle needs little introduction. Certainly I do not feel I need to give you any instructions on how to cultivate them! Despite the fact that nettle can be such a scourge to the gardener, it is an extremely valuable medicinal aid.

First and foremost nettle is a detoxifying herb, eliminating waste products and increasing urine output. It is therefore extremely useful in the treatment of osteoarthritis and indeed any arthritic problems, also gout. It is also particularly helpful where there is poor kidney function and fluid retention.

Nettle helps slow and stop bleeding and therefore is a good remedy for heavy menstrual bleeding. Nettle also has an extremely high iron content. Therefore, not only does it slow bleeding but after chronic blood loss, when anaemia could be present, nettle provides valuable iron – clever stuff!

Nettle is also very helpful in the treatment of hay fever, asthma and for skin conditions such as acne, psoriasis and eczema.

With its high iron content nettle has unquestioning tonic value and can be used as a tasty vegetable very similar to spinach.

Combinations
NETTLE with ELDERFLOWER for hay fever.
NETTLE with PALEMENTO for enlarged prostrate.
NETTLE with CELERY SEED for gout.
NETTLE with BURDOCK and ECHINACEA for acne and other skin conditions.

PARSLEY PIERT

Unlike many herbs in this book, whose origins for medicinal use go back to Roman, Greek and ancient Egyptian times, parsley piert is essentially a British herb. Parsley has a reputation for the treatment of kidney and bladder problems, especially kidney stones. It is particularly helpful where gravel and stones have collected in the bladder and are causing irritation and discomfort and generally obstructing urine flow. It has not been established as to whether parsley actually helps break down the kidney stones but certainly it is very helpful in the treatment of the often distressing symptoms of kidney stones.

Parsley is also very helpful in the treatment of oedema of kidney or liver origin, and is a general, soothing diuretic.

Parsley is very useful in the treatment of cystitis and indeed any recurrent urinary tract infection. It is mildly astringent.

Although not considered one of the greats of herbal medicine, parsley was spoken very highly of by Gerard in the 17th century and should not be dismissed where there are any problems associated with kidneys or bladder.

Combinations
PARSLEY with CORNSILK and BUCHU for cystitis.
PARSLEY with CORNSILK for kidney stones.

PASSIFLORA

Passiflora does exactly what the name suggests, it pacifies! It is a native plant of both North and South America and is now cultivated in Europe, particularly in Italy. Passiflora is a very valuable medicine for tension, anxiety, irritability and insomnia. Its properties as a sedative and tranquilliser are well-established passiflora is the herb to take when life has simply become too much – it will relax and soothe, and stem the panic and over-activity which often occurs when a person is under stress. It will also calm nervousness and over excitability. Although passiflora is a natural tranquilliser, it is totally non-addictive and does not cause any drowsiness. It calms.

Passiflora is sometimes prescribed in cases of convulsion, epilepsy and hysteria. It has an anti-spasmodic action which helps control hypertension, palpitations, period pains and even asthma

It is often used by sufferers of Parkinson's disease, and can be very effective in the treatment of nerve pain – as in neuralgia and shingles. However passiflora remains best known as a remedy for insomnia created by stress and overwork.

Combinations
PASSIFLORA with VALERIAN ROOT for insomnia.
PASSIFLORA with FEVERFEW for migraines and headaches.
PASSIFLORA with CHAMOMILE FLOWERS for irritable bowel syndrome.

PSYLLIUM HUSK

Psyllium husk is a bulk forming laxative and is anti-diarrhoeal. This in itself sounds like a contradiction in terms, but what psyllium husk does is to regularise bowel movements. It bulks up stool weight where diarrhoea is a feature and prevents hard dry stools where constipation is the problem.

For this reason psyllium husk has become a very useful herb for people trying to lose weight or who are on a calorie controlled diet since as well as bulking up the contents of the bowel, psyllium husk has the effect of moving it quickly through the system. Psyllium husk also reduces cholesterol levels which again is a useful tool in the fight against weight problems. Psyllium husk is very helpful in the treatment of irritable bowel syndrome, diverticulitis and haemorroids.

Psyllium husk should be taken with plenty of water, and if you are taking any other drugs or medication, they should be swallowed one hour before psyllium husk.

Combinations
PSYLLIUM HUSK with BOLDO for slimming diets.
PSYLLIUM HUSK with KELP for weight reduction.
PSYLLIUM HUSK with CRANESBILL for haemorroids.
PSYLLIUM HUSK with FENNEL and WILD YAM for irritable bowel syndrome.
PSYLLIUM HUSK with SLIPPERY ELM for intestinal upsets.

RASPBERRY LEAF

Raspberry leaf is recognised as the herb of pregnancy. In the early days of pregnancy, raspberry relieves nausea and helps prevent miscarriage. However, it is probably best known for its properties during the last trimester for preparing the muscles of the womb for birth. It is believed that raspberry leaf stimulates the longtitudinal muscles of the womb and relaxes the cervix, thereby contributing to an easy birth. Let's face it – it's worth trying anything!

Raspberry leaf is very helpful as a remedy for heavy menstrual bleeding and period pains, and is often prescribed for menopausal problems as it is an oestreogenic herb. As raspberry leaf has a high calcium content, it is useful to take during the menopause and beyond, to prevent the onset of osteoporosis.

Raspberry leaf was used in the past as an astringent for the healing and washing of wounds. Today, the astringent quality makes it a useful gargle for relieving sore throats, mouth ulcers and gingivitis. Equally it is valuable as an eyewash in the case of conjunctivitis.

Raspberry leaf taken as an infusion is helpful in the relief of diarrhoea and helps reduce irritability within the bowel – ie as in diverticulitis.

Combinations
RASPBERRY LEAF with BLACK COHOSH and WILD YAM for period pains.
RASPBERRY LEAF with CRANESBILL for diarrhoea.
RASPBERRY LEAF with BLACK COHOSH and SAGE for menopausal problems.

RED CLOVER

Red clover has many attributes but it is most effective in the treatment of the skin. It is an extremely important aid to chronic skin conditions, such as eczema, acne, psoriasis and cold sores, which may refuse to heal. It is particularly associated with children's skin problems and is a safe remedy to use in the case of very young children.

Red clover has a growing reputation in the treatment of cancer. Traditionally it has been used as a drink for cleansing the lymphatic vessels through which cancer is believed to spread. More recently it has proved useful in the reduction of tumours and hard swellings, particularly in the ovaries and breasts.

Being anti-inflammatory, red clover also helps prevent ulceration and is particularly helpful with mouth ulcers and sore throats.

Red clover has also been used to good effect in the treatment of whooping cough and bronchitis, and many years ago in the treatment of tuberculosis. It is an expectorant and anti-spasmodic.

Combinations

RED CLOVER with CHICKWEED OINTMENT for eczema and psoriasis.
RED CLOVER with YELLOW DOCK and NETTLE for chronic skin disease.

ROSEMARY

Rosemary is a herb to raise the spirits! A Mediterranean herb since time immemorial, rosemary was introduced to this country during the 14th century Gerard summed it up by saying it 'comforteth the harte and maketh it merie.'

Rosemary is a stimulant and tonic for both heart and nervous system. It lifts and energises both the mind and body. From the time of ancient Greece onwards, students used rosemary to improve their memory during the taking of exams. I have tried sending my boys off to school exams with a sprig of rosemary, but they were horrified by the suggestion – words like 'naf' and 'sad' ricocheted about. I'll try again for GCSE!

Rosemary also relieves headaches and migraines by improving blood circulation to the scalp, which in turn has the added effect of improving hair growth.

Rosemary encourages recovery from long-term, stressful illness and generally improves debilitating states. In today's stressful world, rosemary can often help people who are not actually ill, in a clinical sense, but simply do not seem to be thriving. Rosemary promotes a more optimistic view of life, which in itself is extremely valuable.

Combinations
ROSEMARY with ST JOHN'S WORT and LEMON BALM for depression.
ROSEMARY with YARROW for 'failure to thrive'.
ROSEMARY with ECHINACEA ROOT for chronic infections.

ST JOHN'S WORT

Extensive research has taken place over the years into the effectiveness of St John's wort as an anti-depressant. Numerous clinical trials were conducted in the last twenty years of the 1900s, and as a result of this research, the British Medical Journal on 8th August 1996 was forced to admit that the evidence for St John's wort activity as an anti-depressant was fairly compelling. While from time to time, St John's wort gets a bad press from medical professionals, the fact is that it works. St John's wort is nature's answer to Prozac. It is an anti-depressant which is neither addictive, nor does it have any awful side effects. In Germany, it is widely used for moderate and mild depression and some enlightened psychiatrists in this country use it on a regular basis.

The attributes of St John's wort do not end with depression, however. St John's wort improves a whole range of nervous problems, such as tension, anxiety, insomnia and the effects of the menopause.

St John's wort is anti-viral and is used in the treatment of hepatitis, flu and recently, it was found to be very effective in treating HIV infection.

It is of little surprise, perhaps, that in the ancient world, as early as the 1st century AD, St John's wort had a reputation for driving away demons – demons in the head one suspects – which proves nothing much changes through the centuries, one way or another.

Warning: There are some prescription drugs which should not be taken with St John's wort. Therefore, do seek advice before combining St John's wort with any medication. St John's wort does make you slightly more susceptible to sunburn, so you may need a higher factor sun cream.

Combinations

ST JOHN'S WORT with BLACK COHOSH for menopausal problems including hot flushes.
ST JOHN'S WORT with DAMIANA for depression linked to nervous exhaustion.
ST JOHN'S WORT with ECHINACEA ROOT and LEMON BALM for viral infections including herpes.

SAGE

Traditionally Sage is associated with old age and has a reputation for encouraging longevity and restoring failing memory. It is often planted on graves and around the church porches as a mark of respect to the elderly deceased!

Sage is mainly seen as a herb for the throat. It is antiseptic and astringent and helps relax the throat – indeed all throat infections respond to sage.

Sage is also used extensively in China for dyspepsia, diarrhoea and irritable bowel syndrome.

Sage has also proved itself to be excellent during the menopause, particularly in reducing hot flushes. How it does this is not understood, but somehow its oestreogenic nature has the effect of reducing sweating and helps the body adapt to hormonal changes.

Sage is also believed to help in the treatment of Alzheimer's disease, as well as general memory lapses.

Combinations
SAGE with AGNUS CASTUS and BLACK COHOSH for the menopause.
SAGE with ECHINACEA for sore throats.
SAGE with ECHINACEA and GINGER ROOT for gastroenteritis.

SAW PALMETTO

Early settlers in the USA claimed their animals grew 'sleek and fat on the fruits of Saw Palmetto.' Certainly this is logical as saw palmetto has the reputation of being a building and strengthening herb, a tonic for general debility and weakness. Early herb books describe it mainly as a man's herb as it has a reputation for improving hormonal disorders and testicular wasting, and acts as a general boost to male sex hormones. It also has the apparent ability to tone up and strengthen the neck of the bladder and reduce obstruction of the bladder by an enlarged prostate gland. However, saw palmetto is also considered a useful tonic for women as well, particularly where there is a failure to thrive.

Saw palmetto is also used for improving urinary flow and is known as a tonic diuretic. It is anti-inflammatory and anti-spasmodic and is therefore very helpful in the treatment of irritable bladder conditions, including cystitis.

Combinations

SAW PALMETTO and NETTLE ROOT for benign prostate enlargement.
SAW PALMETTO with ECHINACEA and WILLOW BARK for prostatitis.
SAW PALMETTO with BUCHU for irritable bladder.
SAW PALMETTO with DAMIANA for impotence.

SKULLCAP

In our workaholic, stressed society, skullcap is re-emerging as the remedy for overwork, stress, nervous tension, anxiety, insomnia, irritability, depression and headaches. This is a seriously useful herb. Skullcap is a 'nervine' remedy which works on both the nervous and the digestive systems. Skullcap is anti-spasmodic and because of this, is also seen as a herb with a 'deeper' action on the nervous system. Skullcap is used for convulsions, epilepsy and hysteria, as well as serious mental illness. Although in the case of these chronic conditions, skullcap is not a treatment in its own right, it has a growing reputation for proving very helpful in serious conditions.

For most of us though, skullcap helps us to cope with life, with panic attacks, with anxiety and all the stresses and strains of modern living. Skullcap also possesses anti-inflammatory action so is often prescribed for inflammatory conditions such as rheumatoid arthritis and muscular tension, both conditions often aggravated by long term stress.

Skullcap is also useful as a general tonic after long term illness, particularly if that illness has resulted in a high level of stress or anxiety.

Combinations
SKULLCAP with CRAMP BARK for menstrual pain.
SKULLCAP with BLACK COHOSH for rheumatoid arthritis.
SKULLCAP with St JOHN'S WORT for depression.
SKULLCAP with VALERIAN for insomnia.
SKULLCAP with CHAMOMILE FLOWERS for nervous digestion.
SKULLCAP with FEVERFEW for migraine.
SKULLCAP with PASSIFLORA for hyperactivity.

SLIPPERY ELM

Slippery elm soothes and relieves – it is a great companion to have through the rigours of life! It is perhaps best known as a 'tummy herb' as it quietens considerably the effects of gastroenteritis, diarrhoea and any form of weakened digestion, perhaps as a result of illness. Within the gut, it soothes away inflammation and will reduce colic and spasms. It also helps problems of the colon such as colitis, irritable bowel syndrome and internal haemorrhoids. Weirdly, as well as easing the effects of diarrhoea, slippery elm is also very helpful for constipation – in other words its job is to regulate the bowel whatever the problem.

Slippery elm is also useful for chest conditions from colds and coughs through to bronchitis, pleurisy and tuberculosis. The powdered bark is particularly good for sore throats. I stress powdered bark because slippery elm bark is seldom sold in pieces – indeed in much of the USA it is against the law to sell slippery elm bark in pieces longer than 1.5 inches. This is because, in the past, slippery elm was used to provoke abortions by inserting long pieces of bark into the cervix – very effective apparently and also very illegal.

Combinations
SLIPPERY ELM with THYME for chronic coughs.
SLIPPERY ELM with CRANESBILL for diarrhoea.
SLIPPERY ELM with CHAMOMILE FLOWERS and FENUGREEK for gastritis and peptic ulcers.

TEA TREE

Tea tree is indigenous to New South Wales, Australia. Its properties have been used by Aboriginal tribes for thousands of years. The oil is found within the cells of the leaves and is renowned for its amazing antiseptic qualities. Tea tree is effectively nature's antiseptic.

Tea tree is also anti-fungal and a germicide. It possesses rejuvenating properties for the skin. For this reason, tea tree has been very much taken up by the cosmetic industry. It can now be found in soaps, shampoo and deodorants and a wide range of skin care products. While this is good, it is important that tea tree should not debased as a tool for the cosmetic industry. It should be valued for its real medical qualities.

Most of the surface problems of the body will benefit from tea tree. Because tea tree is such a versatile plant, it is impossible within the confines of this book to list all the combinations where tea tree would be appropriate. However, tea tree, applied externally, supported by a herb taken internally, is often very effective. For example in the case of acne – tea tree applied to spots externally, with echinacea root taken internally for its anti-bacterial, anti-viral properties, would be an excellent combination.

THYME

Thyme has such a glowing reputation as a culinary herb and is so easy to grow in so many different varieties, that one could be forgiven for overlooking the fact that it is also a very serious medicinal herb and, as such, is I think, generally under appreciated.

Thyme is a particularly good herb for chest infections, whether minor, or serious, such as bronchitis, whooping cough and pleurisy. Combined with lobelia, it is excellent for asthma, particularly in children because not only does thyme have tonic qualities, it is also a gentle sedative.

Thyme is also good with fungal infections and is particularly effective if the fresh leaves are chewed to relieve sore throats.

Externally thyme has many uses – as an infusion it is useful for arthritic and rheumatic aches and pains and should be massaged well into the area. This also applies to sciatica. Because of its ability to remedy fungal infections, thyme is very helpful as a lotion if applied to athlete's foot, thrush, ringworm and lice. I have found that combined with other herbs, thyme is an extremely useful treatment for head lice.

Thyme should also always be viewed as an excellent all round tonic, which is pleasant to taste as a tea. It will greatly improve your 'feel good' factor, thus proving that thyme is as useful in the medicine chest as it is in the kitchen.

Thyme also has a reputation for assisting in the breaking of an alcohol habit, taken either as tea or a tincture.

Combinations
THYME with ECHINACEA and ELECAMPANE for bronchitis and chest infections.
THYME with LOBELIA for asthma.
THYME with TEA TREE, ROSEMARY and LAVENDER for head lice.

TURMERIC

One associates turmeric with curry dishes but it is also an extremely useful medicinal herb. It is used as a blood purifier, it is an anti-oxidant and a bowel stimulant. Turmeric is also an excellent detoxifier and regenerates liver tissue. It also has anti-inflammatory qualities which makes it very helpful for arthritis, skin disorders and asthma. Turmeric has anti-tumor activity and is therefore anti-cancer. Studies have shown that it is one of the strongest free radical scavengers and in addition to its many other properties, turmeric is cholesterol lowering.

Turmeric helps in reducing blood loss both externally and internally so is helpful in a wide range of circumstances – such as the birth of a child, or a nose bleed, or a heavy menstrual cycle. It can be used both internally and externally to heal wounds.

Turmeric capsules are readily available from most health stores but as an alternative, it is such a useful and health giving spice you can simply introduce it more often into your cooking if you have no specific ailment that needs treatment. A number of studies have shown that turmeric does provide a degree of protection against cancer, and its cholesterol lowering activities make it a very useful herb to make a part of your regular diet.

Combinations
TURMERIC with MILK THISTLE and DANDELION for liver conditions.

VALERIAN

Valerian is nature's tranquilliser. With life's increasing stress levels, valerian has never been more popular, and with good cause. While it is a tranquillising and calming herb, valerian's true strength lies in its ability to promote good sleep. Valerian will not only affect the length of sleep but also the quality, encouraging deeper sleep and less frequent waking. The huge benefit is that despite its powers, valerian does not produce drowsiness so that it is quite safe to take it and drive a car or work machinery. Its other major benefit is that unlike many sleeping pills, it is totally non-addictive and there are no apparent side effects. Yet the taking of valerian does have a quite dramatic effect on sleep patterns and often very quickly. Customers come into our shop while on holiday in Cornwall, very often unable to sleep in unfamiliar surroundings and on a different bed. We give them valerian and usually they are back the following day, saying they have immediately had a decent night's sleep.

Valerian should be viewed also as a benefit to those of us who are still awake! If you are a chronic worrier, who cannot switch off after a day's work, then valerian will help to relax you. It is also helpful with all nervous disorders such as panic attacks, sweating and palpitations. Valerian is also used where high blood pressure is caused by stress.

Valerian also has a calming effect on the body as well as the mind. It will relieve muscular problems such as a frozen shoulder, back pain and neck tension. It also eases period pains, asthma, colic and irritable bowel – in other words its calming effect is of benefit to the whole body.

Combinations
VALERIAN with HAWTHORN for high blood pressure linked with stress.
VALERIAN with ST JOHN'S WORT for insomnia and anxiety linked with depression.
VALERIAN with CHAMOMILE for digestive or menstrual cramping pains.

VERVAIN

Vervain is not particularly well known and a rather undervalued medicinal herb. Yet it has great restorative powers especially in relieving nervous tension and stress. It acts as a tonic and while it does have anti-depressant qualities, it is most valuable where nervous exhaustion and anxiety are the chief symptoms. It is the ideal herb to take after a long period of stress or chronic illness and more recently it has been discovered to be very helpful in the treatment of M.E.

Vervain may also be given for relief from asthma, insomnia and headaches/migraine.

In Chinese medicine, vervain is particularly associated with migraine and also with the menstrual cycle, relieving the symptoms of pre-menstrual tension, particularly where irritability is a feature.

Vervain has a particular affinity with both the kidneys and the liver and is helpful where the liver is congested and the patient jaundiced.

Vervain also helps promote the production of milk in nursing mothers.

Combinations
VERVAIN with CHAMOMILE for postnatal depression.
VERVAIN with OATS for liver depression.
VERVAIN with ROSEMARY and THYME for nervous exhaustion.
VERVAIN with AGNUS CASTUS for pre-menstrual syndrome.

WILD YAM

Wild yam is a major food in America, particularly Mexico, with its potato-like fruit. However wild yam has many important medicinal properties and has been around for a long time – not only was it used by early American settlers, but also by the Aztecs!

Wild yam's main therapeutic uses are for arthritis and rheumatism. It has anti-inflammatory and anti-spasmodic powers which make it a very valuable remedy, particularly where hot inflamed joints are concerned. It also helps relax stiff and aching muscles and relieves muscle spasms and pain.

Wild yam also has a justified reputation for relieving menstrual cramps, and for thousands of years was used to relieve both the pain of periods and of childbirth. While the treatment for pain in childbirth has moved on somewhat, wild yam remains very useful for any spasmodic pains, such as menstrual cramps.

Wild yam is also of benefit to the digestive system, particularly the gall bladder when inflamed and also irritable bowel syndrome and diverticulitis. It also has a reputation for being an excellent tonic for the liver.

Combinations

WILD YAM with DEVIL'S CLAW and WILLOW BARK for inflammatory arthritic conditions.
WILD YAM with CAPSCSICUM and BLACK COHOSH for osteoarthritis.
WILD YAM and AGNUS CASTUS for pre-menstrual syndrome.
WILD YAM and FENUGREEK for diverticulitis.

WILLOW BARK

Willow bark has a fascinating history. Widely used as a herbal medicine for centuries, primarily to reduce fever, it was scientifically investigated in the 19th century by a French chemist, Leroux. He extracted the active constituent and named it Salicine. By 1852 this chemical had been produced synthetically and by 1899 was being marketed as a product called ...Aspirin.

As you might expect, the original willow bark mirrors Aspirin in many respects. It eases pain, reduces fever and is anti-inflammatory. It does not however have the blood thinning properties of Aspirin.

Willow bark is used for arthritic problems where it proves to be very effective and is particularly helpful where pain affects the knees, hips and back. Willow bark cannot reverse arthritic problems and usually needs to be combined with other herbs to be most effective, but it is very useful in the treatment of pain and inflammation. Willow bark is also helpful in the treatment of headaches.

As long ago as the 1st century AD, Dioscorides suggested taking willow leaves 'mashed with a little pepper and drunk with wine to relieve lower back pain'. I'm not sure about pepper but the wine sounds good!

Combinations
WILLOW BARK, CELERY SEED and DANDELION LEAF for osteoarthritis and joint pain.
WILLOW BARK with DEVIL'S CLAW and BLACK COHOSH for rheumatoid and other inflammatory arthritis.
WILLOW BARK with WILD YAM and DEVIL'S CLAW for inflamed arthritic conditions.
WILLOW BARK and FEVERFEW for headache and migraine.
WILLOW BARK and BUCHU LEAF for prostates.

WITCH HAZEL

Witch hazel is a woodland tree indigenous to North America. It was once believed to have occult powers – hence presumably its name. Witch hazel is marvellous for inflamed and tender skin, for bruises, cuts, sprains and swellings. It has the effect of tightening up the proteins in the skin, across the surface of cuts and abrasions, therefore drawing the skin together. For this reason it is very good for sagging skin, which is why it is now used extensively in the cosmetic industry. It is also useful in the treatment of varicose veins.

Witch hazel has a long association with eye problems. Distilled witch hazel water makes a very good eye wash for tired, bruised or inflamed eyes. It is also helpful in the treatment of conjunctivitis.

Witch hazel is also useful in the treatment of haemorrhoids, and will control diarrhoea and ease the symptoms of dysentery, if taken internally.

Combinations
WITCH HAZEL with ECHINACEA for weeping skin infections.
WITCH HAZEL with MARIGOLD for inflamed skin.
WITCH HAZEL distilled with ROSE WATER as a skin tonic.

WORMWOOD

Wormwood is primarily a herb of the digestive system. It is extremely effective for those suffering from an under-active or weak digestion. By aiding the increase of stomach acid and saliva production, it aids digestion and increases the body's ability to resist infection. Wormwood also helps stimulate bile, which in turn relieves symptoms such as bloating and burping. In general terms wormwood strengthens the whole digestive activity and is of great benefit, after a prolonged illness, in helping the body's return to full vitality. Wormwood is also a support to the liver and aids depression, often originating from poor liver function. It will improve poor appetite and bad breath and reduces nausea and vomiting.

Externally wormwood is a very good insecticide and insect repellent. Over many centuries, wormwood branches were used to line drawers to ward off moths. With our increasing understanding as to the damage of modern insecticides, both to us and to our environment, an infusion of wormwood makes a very safe and useful insect spray around the house.

Combinations
WORMWOOD with GOLDEN SEAL, ECHINACEA and GINGER for gastrointestinal infections.

YARROW

Yarrow's Latin name is derived from that of the Greek hero of the Iliad, Achilles. According to mythology, Achilles healed the wounds of his fellow soldiers with yarrow and certainly the herb has been used in the treatment of wounds for thousands of years.

Today, yarrow is valued for its action in colds and influenza, for lowering temperatures and for relieving catarrh and the general build up of mucous.

Yarrow is also helpful, and often prescribed, for cardiovascular complaints and for relieving high blood pressure or thrombosis.

Yarrow is often given in the treatment of colic, diarrhoea, dysentery and stomach cramps.

Harking back to the days of Achilles, yarrow has excellent blood clotting powers The herb is particularly renowned for stopping nosebleeds – fresh leaves can be inserted into the nostrils to stop the bleeding. With this in mind, yarrow tea is reputed to be very helpful in stopping both internal and external bleeding and like so many herbs, it is for its regulatory powers that it is best known – in others words while on one hand, it aids blood clotting, it will also prevent blood clots in the wrong place - ie varicous veins or thrombosis.

Combinations
YARROW with ST JOHN'S WORT for inflamed joints.
YARROW with PEPPERMINT or HYSSOP for chesty colds.

A comprehensive range of herbal medicines, remedies, tinctures, and ointments are available from the **Halzephron Herb Farm** shops in Truro and St Ives. There is plenty of helpful advice on hand. Details as follows:-

TRURO

Halzephron Herb Farm

Lemon Street Market, Truro, Cornwall TR1 2PN
(at the bottom of Lemon Street, near the cinema)

Shop opening hours: 9am – 5pm Monday to Saturday
Closed on Sundays

ST IVES

Halzephron Herb Farm

62, Fore Street, St Ives, Cornwall TR26 1HW
(at the harbour end of Fore Street)

Shop opening hours   10am – 5pm Monday to Saturday
11am – 4pm Sundays between Easter
& Christmas

MAIL ORDER

Telephone: 01736 791891

Fax: 01736 794514

Web: www.halzherb.com